YOUR KNOWLEDGE HAS VALUE

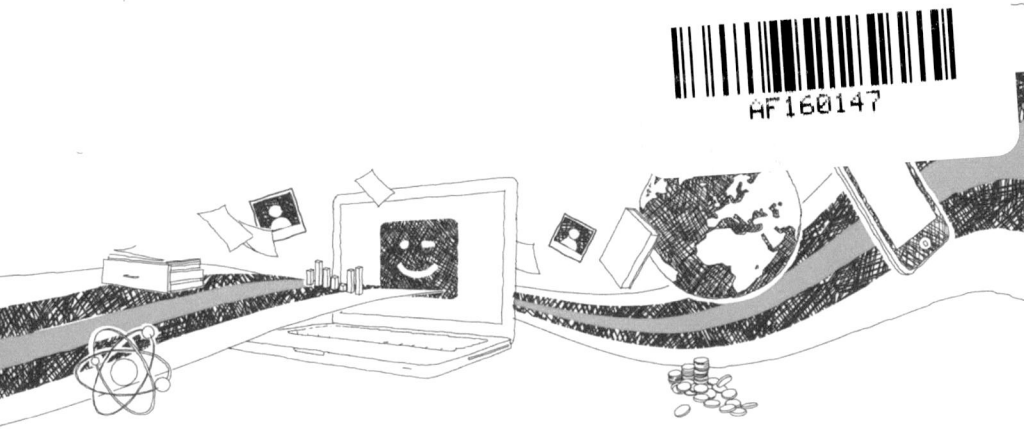

- We will publish your bachelor's and master's thesis, essays and papers

- Your own eBook and book - sold worldwide in all relevant shops

- Earn money with each sale

Upload your text at www.GRIN.com
and publish for free

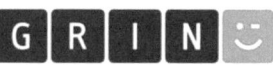

Bibliographic information published by the German National Library:

The German National Library lists this publication in the National Bibliography; detailed bibliographic data are available on the Internet at http://dnb.dnb.de .

This book is copyright material and must not be copied, reproduced, transferred, distributed, leased, licensed or publicly performed or used in any way except as specifically permitted in writing by the publishers, as allowed under the terms and conditions under which it was purchased or as strictly permitted by applicable copyright law. Any unauthorized distribution or use of this text may be a direct infringement of the author s and publisher s rights and those responsible may be liable in law accordingly.

Imprint:

Copyright © 2018 GRIN Verlag, Open Publishing GmbH
Print and binding: Books on Demand GmbH, Norderstedt Germany
ISBN: 9783668623071

This book at GRIN:

https://www.grin.com/document/388558

Patrick Kimuyu

Integration of Theory with Practice. Leukemia Case Reflection

GRIN - Your knowledge has value

Since its foundation in 1998, GRIN has specialized in publishing academic texts by students, college teachers and other academics as e-book and printed book. The website www.grin.com is an ideal platform for presenting term papers, final papers, scientific essays, dissertations and specialist books.

Visit us on the internet:

http://www.grin.com/

http://www.facebook.com/grincom

http://www.twitter.com/grin_com

Integration of Theory with Practice- Leukemia Case Reflection

Name: Patrick Kimuyu

Inhaltsverzeichnis

Introduction 2
Extended Discussion of Perspectives 3
   Pathophysiology 3
   Relevant Pharmacology 5
   Inter-Professional Roles in Patient Centered Care 6
   Psychosocial Issues 7
   Relating Knowledge to Clinical Practice 7
Conclusion 9
References 10

Introduction

In nursing practice, practical skills are essential. It is through practical approaches that learners, as well as practicing nurses apply theoretical knowledge to improve patients' outcome. This is the principal goal of nursing interventions. However, the success of nursing interventions depends on the professional competence of the nurses providing care. It is evident that the level of competence varies among nurses, more or less the same as it is the case with intelligence. Nevertheless, all nurses, as well as other healthcare professionals are expected to demonstrate their potential for giving healthcare services to patients efficiently. This explains why all professionals in healthcare to integrate knowledge and practical skills. This was demonstrated in the simulation activity that involved providing nursing interventions to Jenny, a leukemia patient. Jenny, a 10 year old girl had been diagnosed with leukemia. Six months after her diagnosis with leukemia, she suffered pneumonia that led to her hospitalization for 10 days, after which she was discharged home with home care support services and the palliative care team. During her hospitalization, she received treatment in which nursing interventions were adopted to address the underlying conditions, in order to improve the patient's health and quality of life. For instance, our group offered nursing care to Jenny including administering Ceftriaxone 650Mg BD IV during the simulation session. In this case scenario, several of theoretical perspectives were required. Therefore, this critical reflection will discuss four key theoretical perspectives: pathophysiology, relevant pharmacology, inter-professional roles in patient centered care, and psychosocial issues related to the case scenario, and demonstrate the relationship between theoretical concepts and clinical practice.

Extended Discussion of Perspectives

Pathophysiology

Understanding the pathophysiology of a given condition serves as the key approach to treatment interventions. Ideally, pathophysiology determines the form of intervention that is required to address the issues involved. One of the most important aspects of understanding pathophysiology is to enable healthcare professionals to understand different aspects of diseases. For instance, healthcare practitioners, as well as, medical students understand why diseases develop in the human body with respect to human anatomy. They also learn how diseases develop, as well as how their clinical manifestations appear. These help in the prognosis of a given disease or health condition. Moreover, an extended understanding on the pathophysiology of diseases enables nurses, as well as, other healthcare practitioners to understand the fundamental mechanisms involved in the pathogenesis of diseases. According to theory, different diseases exhibit different mechanisms. Some diseases exhibit neural mechanisms and others exhibit humoral mechanism. On the other hand, diseases can exhibit cellular mechanism or molecular mechanism.

In this case scenario, understanding on the pathophysiology of pneumonia, that was the main reason for hospitalization, as well as, the pathophysiology of leukemia, the underlying condition was paramount. Jenny was diagnosed to have been infected with *Haemophilus influenzae* as the etiological agent for pneumonia. Therefore, it is apparent that Jenny's pneumonia was caused by an extrinsic factor. *Haemophilus influenzae* infested the upper airways and colonized the lung parenchyma. As a result, bacterial pneumonia developed due to the impaired local defenses, a phenomenon that is related to leukemia disease, deteriorated health status of the patient, and virulence of the infecting *Haemophilus influenzae*. This infection in the pulmonary system led to acute inflammation of the airways. This inflammation was caused by the filling of air spaces with neutrophils that migrated out of capillaries (Kamangar 2015). Therefore, treatment was aimed at eradicating the causative agent that was responsible for the pathophysiology and restoring normal pulmonary function.

On the other hand, there was also the underlying pathophysiology related to leukemia. Leukemia begins with the occurrence of a clone of malignant cells during lymphoid cellular maturation. In most cases, rearrangement of the DNA in leukemic cells occurs due to external factors. Some of these factors are chemicals, ionizing radiation and alkylating drugs. On the other hand, internal factors such as genetic abnormalities including chromosomal mutations are responsible for DNA changes related to the formation of malignant lymphatic cells. It is suggested that chromosomal rearrangements cause alterations in the regulation and structure of cellular oncogenes. In the case Jenny, the cause of leukemia appears to be caused by chromosomal abnormalities. In lymphocytic leukemia, the sequence of genes is altered by chromosomal translocations that place genes responsible for normal cellular proliferation and activation next to those genes that regulate the synthesis of immunoglobulin proteins, primarily the light chain and heavy chain immunoglobulin proteins. Therefore, these genetic alterations lead to lymphoblast proliferation, resulting to the failure of the bone marrow. The outcome of these hematopoietic mechanisms causes pancytopenia due to the expansion of immature cells in the bone marrow. It is also believed that normal hematopoietic process is inhibited by secretions produced by the abnormal lymphatic cells. Further proliferation of lymphoblasts in the bone marrow leads to the spilling of abnormal cells into the circulation. In addition, abnormal cells infiltrate other organs including the eyes, the spleen and the liver, and opportunistic infection serves as one of the core manifestations (Wu 2015). This explains why Jenny presented with pneumonia following diagnosis with leukemia.

From the nursing perspective, the rationale for addressing the pathophysiology of the disease was to relief the symptoms associated to pneumonia. In addition, focus on the pathophysiology of leukemia was necessary in order to assess the progression of the condition.

Relevant Pharmacology

The second perspective involved in this case scenario was the pharmacology related to the disease. In practice, it is apparent that understanding of pharmacology related to different diseases forms the basis for effective therapeutic treatment of diseases. It is reported that efficacy, safety and tolerability of medications by patients determines their clinical usefulness. Therefore, understanding on the intended drug indications and the involved pharmacokinetics, side effects and the associated potential adverse reactions serves paramount relevance (Berger & Iyengar 2011). In practice, antibiotic therapy in the treatment of *Haemophilus influenzae* involves the use of beta-lactamase, as well as non beta-lactamase drugs. Amoxicillin is the most commonly used non beta-lactamase drug that is recommended as first-line therapeutic agent. However, fluoroquinolone, azithromycin, doxycycline, and clarithromycin are used as alternative antimicrobials for the treatment of *Haemophilus influenzae* infection. On the other hand, second or third generation cephalosporin, beta-lactamase drugs are used as first-line agents for bacterial pneumonia (Kamangar 2015).

On the other hand, the management of leukemia involves the use of several therapeutic agents whose actions are intended to address the underlying symptoms of the disease. Some of these medications include hydrocortisone, maxalon, ibuprofen, and paracetamol.

Ideally, the rationale for engaging pharmacological perspective in the case scenario was to eradicate the bacterial infection that was responsible for pneumonia, and enhancing the management of leukemia.

Inter-Professional Roles in Patient Centered Care

Inter-professional collaboration is another significant perspective that is involved in patient centered care. From a theoretical approach, inter-professional education is meant to equip students with appropriate skills that will enable them to become inter-professional team members in healthcare. It is believed that inter-professional collaboration enhances the provision of patient centered care; thus improving outcomes. This is so because inter-professional teams bring together different professional skills that meet the complex health needs of patients (Lumague et al. 2008). According to the Institute of Medicine (IOM) observes that inter-professional teams can address the complexity and challenging needs by patients through efficient communication leading to appreciable outcome. For instance, inter-professional teams facilitate the sharing of expertise from different disciplines in designing the most appropriate perspective that lead to the restoration or maintenance of patient's health (IOM 2001). In addition, inter-professional approach improves the patient's outcome through pulling together resources (Barker & Oandasan 2005). In general, inter-professional collaborative practice enhances a synergistic influence of grouped skills and knowledge through extensive communication and decision-making. Ordinarily, inter-professional collaboration in patient centered care enables the team to achieve a common goal because collaborative practice involves several elements that are essential in clinical interventions. Some of the key elements of inter-professional collaborative practice are communication, coordination, responsibility, autonomy, and accountability. In addition, collaborative practice involves mutual trust and respect, assertiveness and cooperation as key elements, and this improves patient outcomes (Bridges, Davidson, Odegard, Maki & Tomkowiak 2011). It is believed that collaborative interactions blends professional cultures leading to the improvement of quality of care offered to patients by the team (Morrison 2007). Therefore, inter-professional collaboration is an essential element in patient centered care. IOM recommends that students are supposed to be engaged in the decision – making process, especially on ways of improving the quality of care (IOM 2011).

The rationale for inter-professional perspective is to improve the patient's quality of care and outcomes through patient centered care.

Psychosocial Issues

Moreover, psychosocial issues require attention, especially in cases involving terminal illnesses such as cancer, diabetes and other terminal illnesses. Patients require psychosocial support, in order to experience an improved quality of life. In practice, patients experience an array of psychosocial issues. For instance, some patients experience anxiety disorder that needs intervention. In terminally-ill patients, issues such as end-of-life decisions and palliative care are essential in improving the patient's quality of life.

Relating Knowledge to Clinical Practice

From a critical perspective, knowledge and clinical practice are related in many aspects. This is why simulation sessions are essential in transforming theoretical knowledge into practice. They provide hands-on experience that is required for professional competence in the clinical practice.

In the case scenario, theoretical knowledge on the pathophysiology of pneumonia and leukemia enabled our team to offer the most appropriate nursing care. For instance, the team applied nursing interventions that were aimed at addressing the symptoms of the disease. One of the most critical interventions undertaken during the simulation to solve the patient's breathing problem was ventilatory support. The team was able to administer supplemental oxygen to the patient, in order to prevent dyspnea leading to recovery. It is worth noting that respiratory support plays a key role in the treatment of bacterial pneumonia (Kamangar 2015).

On the other hand, understanding on the relevant pharmacology was essential in enhancing the success of the simulation session that focused on improving Jenny's outcome. In eradicating the bacterial infection, the team administered Ceftriaxone 650 Mg in 10 ml BD IV. Ceftriaxone is a third generation cephalosporin; thus it was ideal for treating bacterial pneumonia caused by *Haemophilus influenzae*. In addition knowledge on pharmacology enabled the team to assess the efficacy, safety and adverse effects of the choice of antimicrobial therapy. Advanced knowledge was required to understand the use of other medications administered to the patient such as hydrocortisone 70Mg TDS IV, Maxalon 10 Mg, ibuprofen and paracetamol. Hydrocortisone 70Mg TDS IV was meant to reduce pneumonia-caused inflammation, whereas Maxalon 10 Mg controlled its side effects including nausea and vomiting. On the other hand, ibuprofen and paracetamol was used for pain, discomfort and fever relief.

Similarly, inter-professional collaboration enabled the team to offer patient centered care to the patient. For instance, the team coordinated with the doctor to solve treatment complications.

Conclusion

In a brief conclusion, this paper offered a critical reflection on Jenny's case scenario and discussed the relationship between theoretical knowledge and clinical practice. It is apparent that theoretical knowledge is necessary for competence in clinical practice. According to the nursing interventions offered to Jenny, the team demonstrated the significance of understanding the pathophysiology involved, pharmacology and psychosocial issues. More important to note was the element of inter-professional collaboration that enhanced the patient's outcomes. For instance, the administration of Ceftriaxone was meant to eradicate the bacteria, whereas hydrocortisone controlled inflammation related to pneumonia. Moreover, collaborative approaches enabled the team to seek assistance from the doctor, as well as, in making decision of respiratory support. Therefore, it is apparent that theoretical concepts and essential in clinical practice.

References

Barker, K & Oandasan, I 2005, Interprofessional care review with medical residents: lessons learned, tensions aired – a pilot study, *J Interprof Care*, vol. 19, 207–14.

Berger, S & Iyengar, R 2011, Role of systems pharmacology in understanding drug adverse events,*Wiley Interdiscip Rev Syst Biol Med.*, vol. 3 no. 2, 129–135.

Bridges, D, Davidson, R, Odegard, PS, Maki, IV & Tomkowiak, J 2011, Interprofessional collaboration: three best practice models of interprofessional education, *Med Educ Online*, vol. 16, 10.3402/meo.v16i0.6035, viewed 20 September 2015, < http://www.ncbi.nlm.nih.gov/pmc/articles/PMC3081249/ >

IOM [Institute of Medicine], 2011, *The future of nursing: leading change, advancing health*, The National Academies Press, Washington, DC.

IOM, 2001, *Crossing the quality chasm: a new health system for the 21st century*, The National Academy Press, Washington, DC.

Kamangar, N 2015, *Bacterial pneumonia*, viewed 19 September 2015, < http://emedicine.medscape.com/article/300157-overview#showall >

Lumague, M, Morgan, A, Mak, D, Hanna, M, Kwong, J, Cameron, C, Zener, D & Sinclair, L 2008, Interprofessional education: the student perspective. *J Interprof Care*, vol. 20, 246–53.

Morrison, S 2007, Working together: why bother with collaboration? *Work Bas Learn Prim Care*, vol. 5, 65–70.

Wu, L 2015, *Leukemias*, viewed 19 September 2015, < http://emedicine.medscape.com/article/1201870-overview#showall >

YOUR KNOWLEDGE HAS VALUE

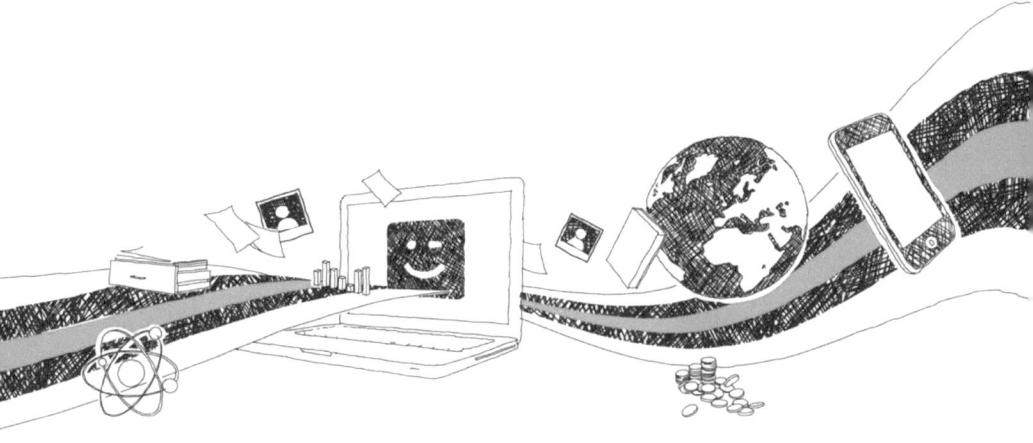

- We will publish your bachelor's and master's thesis, essays and papers

- Your own eBook and book - sold worldwide in all relevant shops

- Earn money with each sale

Upload your text at www.GRIN.com
and publish for free

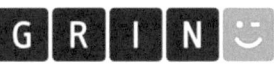